Breathing Miracles

Self-Healing Through Transformational Breath®

Breathing Miracles

Self-Healing Through Transformational Breath®

Kathy M. Smith

Breath Miracles Press

Breathing Miracles
Self-Healing Through Transformational Breath®

Notice to the Reader: This book is intended for informational purposes only. No claims are made as to specific health benefits and it is recommended that persons suffering with mental or physical disease seek the professional or medical treatment of choice. Neither the publisher, author nor the Transformational Breath Foundation may be held responsible for misunderstandings or misuse of the information contained herein. Sessions with a professionally trained Certified Transformational Breath Facilitator™ is recommended before trying any breath session on your own.

Copyright ©2020 by Kathy M. Smith.
All Rights Reserved.
1st Edition published by Breath Miracles Press
ISBN 978-1-7347877-8-8

Editing and manuscript preparation: Stephen Gooby
Foreword: Dr. Judith Kravitz

This book is dedicated to my

Son Ed,

Daughter-in-law Mary,

Grandchildren Ashley and Edward,

And all the love and memories you gift me with!

ACKNOWLEDGMENTS

My deepest gratitude to Dr. Judith Kravitz who introduced so many of us to the gift of Transformational Breath. This gift continually helps me to design a life beyond my wildest expectations. In addition, she gave me the opportunity and the help to create my own miracle.

I am so appreciative and thankful to Stephen Gooby for all his endless guidance, time, and energy in the creation of this miracle. He made it feel real and truly helped to make it a masterpiece.

Thank you to my Uncle Jim Galligan for his help and patience with the endless details of this creation.

I am forever grateful to my incredible fiancé and partner, Buster B. for his never-ending encouragement and support. He was truly instrumental in this becoming a reality

Thank you to my Dad, Mom and siblings Jackie, Frank, Terry, Billy, Tom and Regina for all that I have and continue to learn.

Thank you to my Artist Conference Network family for your ongoing support and encouragement.

Thank you to Ed Smith, for being such an instrumental spiritual teacher in my life and for sharing your wonderful parents, Elliott and Nancy with me.

Thank you to Joan Redding who gifted me with a beautiful friendship and several miracles.

Thank you to all my clients who made this book possible by sharing their experiences.

Thank you to my extraordinary family and friends who are always there for me with support and wisdom.

FOREWORD

by Dr. Judith Kravitz

How would you like to live a life filled with Miracles and magic? What would be possible if you realized that the access key is only a breath away? Are you ready to learn about the greatest gift we have to heal and change our lives?

By reading and taking this book into your heart, you could have a whole new level of feeling alive and a transformed relationship with your Breath.

You will read many miraculous and inspiring stories from Kathy's clients from her twenty years experience as a TBF teacher and practitioner.

Stories of how life changing Miracles occur with simple breathing practices and deep session work.

Kathy shares in a simple comprehensive way how Transformational Breath® works on the physical, mental/emotional and spiritual levels to clear and unify us as multidimensional beings.

She also reveals her moving personal story of how Transformational Breath® lifted her from a life of hardship, trauma, and fear to living a happy, balanced life of helping others.

After working with Transformational Breath® for over 40 years, I have witnessed miracle after miracle from assisting clients to breathe better, use the Breath as a powerful tool for subconscious integration and ultimately take one to deeper expanded states of consciousness.

I am sure you will enjoy reading about some of the many lives and situations that have been transformed with the art of conscious full - connected breathing. Kathy leads us on a joyful adventure of rediscovering the many and amazing gifts of our breath.

Judith is the founder of the Transformational Breath Foundation and the developer of the Transformational Breath® process. She has been leading groups and programs for over 40 years. Author of the popular book, "Breathe Deep, Laugh Loudly", she has worked with 100,000's individually and trained thousands professionally.

CONTENTS

INTRODUCTION 1
WHAT IS TRANSFORMATIONAL BREATH®? 4
WHY DO TRANSFORMATIONAL BREATH®? 6
WHAT ARE MIRACLES? 7
I AM IN CHARGE 9
SELF-EXPRESSION 13
BREAKING THROUGH FEAR 15
HEAL THE BODY 17
CHOOSING LIFE 19
THE UNFOLDING 23
TRUE LOVE 25
CREATE YOUR IDEAL LIFE 27
TRUST 29
SELF-WORTH 31
RECLAIM YOUR SUPERPOWERS 33
SPIRITUAL CONNECTION 35
BREATH IS LIFE 39
CALM INSIDE THE STORM 41
CONCLUSION 45
GLOSSARY 47

Introduction

The challenges of a difficult childhood led to a lifelong search to find something that could help others and myself have more happiness, joy and peace. Yoga, Meditation and Cognitive Therapy helped to a point, but Transformational Breath took it to the next level.

I am compassionately aware that my parents did the best they could with what they knew. We were a sizeable family—seven children—and despite the difficulties they faced dealing with what I realized later were their own unresolved emotional wounds, I know that they loved all of us immensely.

I remember one particular time; I was probably 6 or 7 looking around the living room and thinking, "Oh My God, who is going to take care of these children? They need someone. I need someone."

In the morning I would lie in bed trying to guess what the day was going to be like. Of course, it was dependent on Dad. Good ole' Dad. What kind of a mood was Dad going to wake up in? Was there going to be a full-blown fight with Mom or with one of us? Or maybe he wasn't going to get out of bed that day because he was in a depression; that was worse as he would be home all day long. Dad was a genius level, charismatic, raging alcoholic, and when he quit drinking, the same personality traits applied. That being said, he did believe, and tried to be, the best father he was capable of.

Mom was a beautiful, compassionate, caring, codependent woman who did not have energy to handle the daily responsibilities of being a mother. She was trying to figure out how to take care of all of us and at the same time survive. Both physically and emotionally, Mom was spent. She had survived one nervous breakdown with the promise of another one always just over the horizon. Talk about family drama! Or technically, was this trauma?

I was the second eldest but I felt like I had to come up with something to take care of everything and everyone, but especially my brothers and sisters.

About that time, I stepped into the role of Mother. The only problem was, I was a kid myself. A kid, who was trying to figure out how to save my family. "Let's see, what do I have here," a raging father, a stressed-out mother and me, a kid. Boy, this was so scary I could hardly breathe! Besides feeling pretty alone, I thought how the heck was I going to do this?

After many scary hours, I had an idea.

I'd watch television. All those family shows from "Father Knows Best" to the "Brady Bunch". Wow, there are lots of them with families. I can learn what a parent does to take care of the children. And off I went on my mission. I learned that, at night, you made sure the kids went into a clean bed after a bath in clean pajamas, a book read, teeth brushed and of course, sung to sleep. In the morning, feed them a good breakfast and have them brush their teeth again. Make sure they have clean diapers or undergarments and socks. Oh, and don't forget to comb the clean hair.

Ok, have all that down. Now, how did I take care of myself? Other than doing the aforementioned and my homework, I didn't. I lived in my own little world where it was safe. I could commune with angels and have lots of dreams of what life could be like. I wrote plays, and with paper and crayons, made a theatre with my brothers and sisters as the actors. It was really lots of fun and a way to survive daily life.

How did this affect me? Well, you can imagine, there were lots and lots of fears, but I also acquired a lot of strength.

Since I have learned Transformational Breath, I feel that regardless of what happens in life, I have a tool to help me cope. I remember feeling like I could fly after I spent a week doing a Transformational Breath Seminar. After each Transformational Breath session, I would feel like the emotional baggage that I had been carrying for so long was released and I felt lighter and lighter. I was aware of being more present (not regretting the past or worrying about the future) than I had ever experienced. I felt happy in every cell of my body.

I do Transformational Breath on most mornings to set the vibration (a positive vibe) for my day. Life is so much easier. Transformational Breath makes life more of an adventure than a challenge.

My intention is to continue to do my work so that I can be more present and loving in every aspect of my life and to be the best Mom, Mother-In-Law, MeMom to my family and Partner in my relationship.

What Is Transformational Breath®?

Transformational Breath is a dynamically powerful technique of consciously directed breathing. It is an easy-to-learn method that was first developed by Dr. Judith Kravitz in the late 1970's and has gained international acceptance as a powerful, alternative healing technique for the body, mind and spirit.

Transformational Breath works on three levels: The Physical, Mental/Emotional and Spiritual.

On the Physical level, Transformational Breath relieves tension and stress. On the Physical level, it aims to provide more energy, in part by opening up restrictive breathing patterns. It helps the body to come into balance. It supports the healing of different ailments or disease by stimulating the natural healing powers of the mind/body system.

On the Mental level, Transformational Breath helps to dissolve limiting beliefs, thereby achieving peace and expanding creativity.

On the Emotional level, Transformational Breath integrates repressed patterns held in the subconscious and the body and can help the body resolve any kind of trauma, freeing one to experience new levels of love and joy.

On the Spiritual level, Transformational Breath can bring about changes on higher levels that cascade through one's being. For instance, changes in the emotional self will in some way manifest in changes in the physical. This is part of the holistic model.

While there are some similarities, Transformational Breath differs from the breathing exercises one uses in yoga and meditation. In yoga, one may practice any of several pranayama breathing exercises, each with a particular purpose that is different than the full circular breath that Transformational Breath uses.

As for meditation, while there are different styles, most do not involve dynamic breathing. They are more about focusing the mind. Yet, at the end of a Transformational Breath session, most people report feeling that they are in a meditative state of deep peace.

Why Do Transformational Breath®?

- If you would like to reduce or possibly address any physical symptoms in the body ...stress, pain, illness, disease.
- If you need or would like to increase the energy in your body.
- If you struggle with depression or anxiety.
- If you feel lost in your life and need direction or purpose.
- If you would like to reduce stress in your life.
- If you would like to be more creative.
- If you would like to be more confident.
- If you would like to be more secure in yourself.
- If you need help with addictive patterns.
- If you would like to bring to the surface suppressed emotions.
- If you would like to resolve childhood traumas.
- If you would like to accomplish more in your life.
- If you would like to exceed your own expectations in your life.
- If you would like to learn how powerful you truly are.
- If you would like more abundance in your life.
- If you would like more love in your life.
- If you would like better relationships in your life.
- If you want to be happier.
- If you would like a deeper spiritual connection.
- If you need healing of any kind on any level.
- If you would like to learn how to create miracles in your life.

Transformational Breath may help.

What Are Miracles?

A surprising and welcome event that is not explicable by natural or scientific laws and is therefore considered to be the work of a divine agency.

A highly improbable or extraordinary event, development, or accomplishment that brings very welcome consequences.

An amazing product or achievement, or an outstanding example of something.[1]

BELIEVE IN MIRACLES

Each story here has its own miracle... some big... some small, some inexplicable by scientific laws, and some amazing and or extraordinary.

While each miracle is unique to that person, they share Transformational Breath as a healing tool that gives them the ability to bring about any changes that are important to their lives.

The following fourteen stories share how Transformational Breath sessions helped individuals ease anxiety, eliminate physical pain, make more money, attain new jobs, and became more creative, confident and secure with themselves. The names are not real but the miracles are.

---

[1] definitions from Lexico.com / Oxford English Dictionary

1.

I Am In Charge

When Rafaela started to work with Transformational Breath, she was deeply into *victim consciousness*[1]. She described herself as completely broken and totally wrung out from life. She felt overwhelmed, abandoned, and lived in chronic fear. Hearing about her childhood trauma explained so much of the repeated patterns in her life. One of the beautiful aspects of Transformational Breath is how quickly large chunks of trauma can get integrated in a session and start to dramatically improve the quality of a person's life.

Dr. Henry Smith-Rohrberg, American psychotherapist and advocate of Transformational Breath stated, "One Transformational Breath session is equivalent to about two years of psychotherapy."[2] Analyzing and optimizing Rafaela's breath pattern will bring about the desired results without having to relive what created the imbalance to begin with.

Consider that the way we breathe is how we live our life. As we restrict our breathing, and dampen and repress our emotional responses, we are likewise restricting our lives. By focusing our minds and directing our intention behind the breath, we open ourselves to a more expansive, healthy life experience. This is what Transformational Breath can do for us and what it eventually did for Rafaela.

The first thing I observed in Rafaela's breathing was tightness at the base of the sternum; an area called the

---

[1] A state of consciousness in which we deny personal responsibility for events that happen in our lives or the feelings we experience. We have a belief that the world is against us and we are innocent targets of other people's actions or behavior.

[2] A testimonial on Transformational Breath provided to, and shared by, Judith Kravitz.

surrender point[3]. This might prevent her from having a full diaphragmatic breath. When we release the tension in this area it may help to resolve the conflict between the *personal will* and the *higher will*. Rafaela experienced low-level anxiety on a regular basis. When we corrected the tension and the surrounding tightness, she was much calmer and felt so much less reactive to life. Rafaela also stated that she felt more balanced between what her heart and her head wanted.

At this time, Rafaela feels spiritually connected and deeply trusts her life and its process. She has resolved so much trauma and tension in her body that she feels like a totally different person. She is self-empowered and full of self-love. She has created a new life beyond her wildest expectations; a life that includes a life-partner willing to be a father to her daughter, a new home in California, and an opportunity to be financially supported if she chooses to follow a new career path.

Rafaela's Miracle

A life beyond her wildest imagination!

---

[3] A bodymapping point located beneath the sternum around the *xiphoid process* (bony protrusion) that is usually easy to feel or palpate. Bodymapping is a technique using pressure on various points on the body that are associated with specific emotional content. Releasing tension in these points can assist us in releasing emotional repressions or physical tensions.

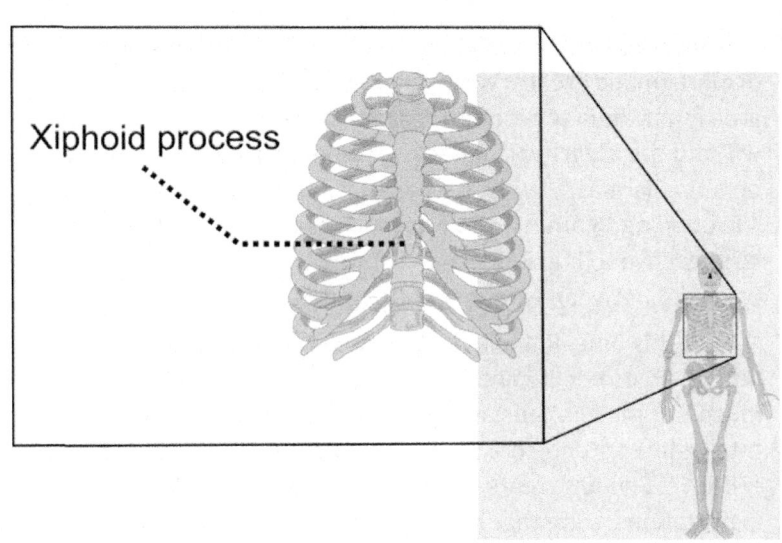

2.

Self-Expression

When Michael first came to me, he was depressed, anxious and felt unable to be his authentic self in his life. For years, Michael had been using anti-depressant and anti-anxiety medicines to cope. He was ready to let these medicines go if he could find a way to have a happy peaceful life without them. Upon observing his breathing pattern, I noticed that he was not able to get breath in his lower abdomen (indicating that he had a hard time staying present in his life and certainly embracing life.)

Transformational Breath uses *Bodymapping to identify and work on various points on the body that correlate with physical tensions and emotional suppressions.* As I applied pressure to these points to help Michael develop a full circular breath, he seemed to come alive with excitement about his life. This is because he was accessing old emotions, traumas, mental patterns etc., and seemingly transforming them from a rather muted expression into something more vibrant and optimistic. We feel this leads to permanent resolution.

I was further guided during one of his sessions to address his diet. I referred him to a clinical nutritionist who found that he was sensitive to gluten and it would be important to eliminate that, and sugar, to fully support the body. Our breathing practice is but one essential aspect of a well-rounded health regimen.

At first, Michael came to me three times a week for 30 days to establish a new way of being and then less frequently as he progressed. It took us a few months for him to reach the point of needing his anti-anxiety meds only once in a while - and then finally not at all. He continues to use

Transformational Breath and watches his diet to maintain these changes.

Michael's Miracle

To be off medication after 25 years!

3.

Breaking Through Fear

Ariel was really surprised at the huge emotional release she experienced and how she felt in her *bodymind*[1] after her first Transformational Breath session. She knew she'd found a way to work with the plans she had for her life. Her intention for that session was to help with the anxiety and worry that she experienced daily.

Upon meeting Ariel, I saw that she was very nervous and ungrounded. After sharing some of her life story, one of her challenges was how inadequate she felt in relation to her sister who she saw as perfect in all areas of her life. Ariel felt that others also perceived that.

When I started to work with Ariel's body, she did not have much movement in her abdomen. When we get the breath into that area, we find it helps to ground us, strengthen our personality, will, and creativity because it permits access to and clearing of the subconscious mind.

As Ariel started to breathe into this area, she had an emotional release and an awareness of how much self-judgment and doubt she had. We worked with a full and easy pattern and introduced *toning*[2] as needed while she continued her session. Continuing this pattern helped her to maintain awareness of her energy and thoughts as they arose in her consciousness. The relaxing body and the letting go of so much held emotion was a beautiful thing to observe.

---

[1] An approach to understanding the relationship between the human body and the mind in seeing them as a single integrated unit (Wikipedia).

[2] Using our vocal expression (the power of sound) to help release or move energy in the body during the breath session.

Ariel is much more confident in herself and her abilities in her work. She is more present in life than ever before. She no longer compares herself to her sister. She feels like the Transformational Breath calms yet energizes her at the same time.

"It is hard to put into words exactly how I feel afterwards and I don't know how it works, I just know I feel really good."

One special thing about Transformational Breath is that we don't have to know exactly what is being held in the body or to analyze anything but the breath pattern. By modifying the breath pattern we get the body to release what is holding us back which, in turn, allows us to break through the confinement of fear.

Ariel's Miracle

She feels much more present in her life and has tremendous confidence about herself and her abilities!

4.

Heal The Body

Seraphina originally came to me because she had been diagnosed with multiple autoimmune disorders. She believed in a functional medical approach, one that combined holistic and western medicine, and wanted to see what holistic options I could offer.

One of my suggestions was to do some Transformational Breath sessions to address any buried emotions that might be the seed cause of the symptoms.

Although Seraphina was a bit skeptical, she agreed to give it a try. At her first session, she mentioned that in addition to the autoimmune disorders, she had an ongoing severe pain in her right hip that multiple chiropractic and massage sessions had not helped. She could barely put her foot down without a burning pain shooting through her hip.

I guided Seraphina into a full *circular breath, where inhalation and exhalation are connected with no pause between breaths, while breathing into the abdomen and upper chest*. After some toning, she soon had a memory surface of the night her parents told the family they were separating and that her father was moving out. Seraphina was just about seven years old at the time and although she didn't understand what it all meant, she remembered she was angry but hadn't said a word about it to anyone. She just unconsciously repressed the emotions in her body.

She also recalled that not long after her parents separated, her dad met and married her stepmother who had two daughters. One of the daughters was close in age to Seraphina. Because their father was not in the picture, Seraphina's dad became the active father to them and had, according to her, neglected his own daughter. (She recalled her father telling her how *he* was resentful towards his own mother for doing the same thing to him). As she continued to breathe, Seraphina started to get in touch with the resentment and anger she had toward her father. She expressed these feelings as part of her session and as it progressed she started to feel lighter. When Seraphina stood up, the hip pain that she'd felt for months was gone and hasn't returned.

Also, her autoimmune issues are in remission and although she found that her diet played a big part in that, I feel that Transformational Breath was essential to her resolution. In fact, Transformational Breath should be a part of a complete holistic approach.

In Transformational Breath, when we have a full circular breath, we have more energy and support for the body's natural healing abilities. This breathing process also helped Seraphina heal the dual traumas of having her parents split up, and then not having her dad around either. These feelings were old, unexpressed emotions that were stored on a cellular and subconscious level. By continuing to breathe through all the memories that were coming up along with the emotions, Seraphina was able to integrate the lower vibration thoughts and feelings of anger and resentment and permanently transmute them into a higher energy form of love and forgiveness.

Seraphina continued to come back for a period of time so that she could eventually have a better relationship with her father and her stepsisters. By working through different layers, Seraphina was able to gain understanding and compassion for her father and realized that her stepsisters needed him as much as she.

Seraphina's Miracle
Months of chronic hip pain - disappeared!

5.

Choosing Life

Daniel is an 85 year-old client who lost his wife to cancer three years before coming to me. She was truly his soulmate, lover, and friend; it was a huge loss for him. He couldn't imagine his life without her.

He had a son from a previous marriage and a stepson and stepdaughter from the later marriage. They were great adult children and very attentive, but it wasn't enough. Daniel was lonely and felt lost.

He had lived a very full life himself. He had been fully engaged in his work, his marriage, and in his community. And although he was well known and loved, he truly did not want to be in this world anymore.

Daniel initially came to me for *Reiki*, a modality often described as hands-on-healing in which a practitioner places hands lightly on or over a patient's body to facilitate the healing process, and other energy work that I combine together. He loved his sessions. He would feel much better for a period of time, but it wouldn't sustain him.

A few months later he ended up in the hospital for an arterial stent and a triple bypass surgery. Could it be that he felt so broken-hearted that he manifested these symptoms unconsciously? I started to introduce him to Transformational Breath a little at a time to see how he would receive it. He loved it!

We began the session with an *Intention*[1] of what he would like to create in his life. Daniel's intention was, "I feel

---

[1] What we would like to have happen as a result of participating fully in the breath session. This would be something positive and empowering.

peace and joy in my life." Because of his physical issues, we decided that the best thing for him would be to combine the energy session with the breathwork.

Part of the Transformational Breath session entails bodymapping[2], working on different points of the body that correlate with physical tensions and emotional suppressions. Since I knew that Daniel had the issues with his heart (stent, bypass), and emotional issues (grief), I applied light pressure to different points across his chest. The first point was to release some physical tension from the surgeries and, second, to encourage him to allow feelings to surface. This gives the feelings an opportunity to be entrained from a lower vibration (grief) to a higher vibration (joy) through the action of our specific breath pattern. I also applied pressure to the area directly underneath the navel. This could possibly address the feelings of not wanting to be alive anymore, thus helping him to desire to more fully participate in life.

I wasn't quite sure what results we would have doing it this way (splitting my focus between energy balancing movements and breath points), but it was worth a try. Daniel really liked the results and they were visible on his face after the session. Taking this approach took us longer to integrate everything, but I believed moving in a positive direction was the most important thing.

On one particular day, not too long after we started this process, Daniel came in feeling very depressed. During our session it wasn't long before Daniel went off mentally to integrate some emotions that had surfaced. He was gone for several minutes. It would appear that he was sleeping and woke screaming, "No, not yet" "I'm not ready" "I can't leave him [his dog]" "NO, NO, NO". I had him open his eyes so that

---

[2] Technique that uses pressure on various points of the body which are associated with specific emotional content. Putting pressure on these points and breathing can assist us in releasing emotional repressions or physical tensions.

he could see where he was. When he realized where he was, he started to get quite emotional and share his experience. He said he had a choice. He felt that he could have left his body permanently if he'd wanted, but he remembered his dog and decided he wasn't going to depart just then. But as Daniel was sitting up, he realized how much power he truly had by being able to leave his body and he was enthralled with the understanding that when it was time, his transition would be easy. The next time I saw Daniel, he was feeling better and decided to "stick around for a while more".

Daniel has moved out of the house that he shared with his wife and bought another. He's decided that he's going to move into the next chapter of his life, with the intention of meeting someone special.

Daniel's Miracle
To go from wanting to die to starting life all over at 85!

6.

The Unfolding

When I first met Gabriel in early 2017, he was going through a tough period in his personal life. He described it as his own learned hopelessness. He was constantly focusing on how dissatisfied he was with himself and his life. He sincerely believed that he was a product of circumstances and had no control over them. He also wanted to make more money, travel more, get a promotion or change jobs, and to feel safe enough to be his authentic self at all times. Gabriel had tried other integrative approaches intended to develop present moment awareness and emotional growth but with limited success.

Gabriel wanted to work with Transformational Breath to see if it could help him shift to a new way of being. He was so committed that he was willing to travel two-and-a-half hours for his appointments, which he did regularly.

As I observed Gabriel's breathing in our first session, I saw that he was unable to breathe into his lower abdomen or stay present in his body (Being fully present means having your focus, your attention, your thoughts and feelings all fixed on what is happening in the body)

I pressed three different points on his body that correlate with various emotions (remember *bodymapping*). One relates to the ability to stay present in the body (i.e. below the navel) and the two others relate to the acceptance and expression of self- empowerment (i.e. under the ribs on the left and right sides). As we did this, it allowed him to integrate lower vibration feelings (fear, insecurity, anger, and resentment) to higher vibrations (courage, security, trust, love, joy, acceptance) and to get a clearer and more loving view of himself.

I also used a fuller and slower breath pattern to send maximum energy throughout his body and to loosen and integrate the suppressed patterns that were contributing to his dissatisfaction and disempowerment.

A key awareness Gabriel made was how much he was out of touch with his own personal power and how that was limiting his life in every area. As he embraced more and more of his own personal power, so many positive experiences started to unfold.

To date, Gabriel has surpassed all but one of his goals, and he has made progress with that. He continues to deepen his understanding of who he is, what he is capable of, and what he really wants in life. He is able to be present with self and continues to move beyond the fear, anger, and grief that he felt was eating him up. By developing a capacity to respond to his experiences instead of reacting and diving into the drama, he's able to take more action and be more loving towards self most of the time.

Gabriel has manifested many things in his life and now makes an amount of money that he once considered ridiculous for – "Someone like him". He is truly aware of how much power he has in creating his perfect life and what it takes to let it unfold and flourish.

Gabriel's Miracle

To make money that he once considered ridiculous for "someone like him"!

7.

True Love

Angelique started out as a massage client to help with anxiety and pain in her body. I would frequently talk about Transformational Breath and how it could help not only with the anxiety, but also with the physical pain issues. She had also struggled for years – unsuccessfully - to feel validated and appreciated in her marriage, and to feel like an equal partner.

She finally gave up trying so hard to get her needs met and instead chose to go along with whatever and however her husband wanted things to be. Angelique felt herself getting more and more shutdown and emotionally suppressed. She decided to focus on having children instead. She struggled for years to get pregnant and eventually, after fertility treatments, had two children by age 37.

As happy as she was to have her children, her marriage continued its decline. Finally, after suffering a heart attack at 39, and having several conversations with me about her marriage difficulties, she decided to give Transformational Breath a try.

We worked together for several months on clearing the unresolved emotions that needed to be integrated in the heart area. We also addressed the points on the body that correlated with receiving and expressing her power. She started to feel that what she had to say mattered and that it was safe to express herself regardless of her husband's reaction. She was feeling stronger and more confident. She believed she deserved to be respected, honored, and loved, and she understood that it had to begin with how she treated herself. She knew that her husband was not in agreement and after numerous attempts to work things out, Angelique made the decision to split up.

Angelique said that this was the most agonizing decision she'd ever made and even harder to follow through with. Yet she knew it was the best thing for her and her children.

Angelique lives in her empowered self and continues to evolve using Transformational Breath as her main tool. She decided not to date anyone for a year after the split so that she would be really clear on how to love and treat herself well first.

Angelique has since met someone who feels like a true partner and best friend and is planning to remarry.

Angelique's Miracle

To truly understand what loving herself feels like!

8.

Create Your Ideal Life

When Charmeine first came for a Transformational Breath session she shared how overwhelmed and exhausted she felt in life.

In 2011, her husband committed suicide, and in 2014, one of her three daughters attempted suicide as well. Another daughter had been diagnosed as anorexic since she was 16 and, as if that wasn't enough emotional stress, Charmeine had a huge financial commitment with her third daughter who was away at college.

Charmeine herself was in a high powered, demanding job with a rigid work schedule. She had no recovery time for herself.

She knew she needed to make a shift, but was not entirely clear on what to do. Nevertheless, Charmeine also knew that she needed to pay close attention to her thought process and how that contributed to her overwhelm. Instead of focusing on what wasn't working, Charmeine started to focus on the changes she wanted to bring about.

At each Transformational Breath session, Charmeine would make an intention as to what she would like to manifest in her life. Working with different points on Charmeine's body and addressing elements of her breathing pattern, we moved toward a full circular breath that would help bring about her heart's desires.

Charmeine was shut down in the chest area where we usually hold onto grief and sadness. As she breathed into this zone and began to integrate traumas she had experienced, Charmeine started to feel lighter and clearer on how she wanted to move forward in her life. She also started to feel more alive and energetic. Each session not only bought

Charmeine closer to a plan of action for her future, but further to a deeper loving connection with herself. She has let go of thoughts and beliefs that no longer serve her and replaced them with more self-empowering ways of thinking.

Charmeine decided that she wanted to retire from her job after 30-some years of service and start in a new direction. She also encouraged her children to begin supporting themselves starting with getting their own homes (all are in their 20's).

Charmeine has retired from her job with an impressive severance package, finished massage therapy school, and is close to finishing her training as a Life Coach.

She is in a new love relationship that is very fulfilling and enjoyable. Charmeine's son has bought his own condo and her daughters are solidifying plans to be on their own. Charmeine is truly living in her power and is creating her life exactly the way she wants it.

Charmeine's Miracle

To have created a life that allows her time to rest, recharge and have fun without financial worries as she decides a future absent of stress or tension!

9.

Trust

The first time I met Mary, a native of Scotland, she was living in New York City on a work visa. She was enthralled with Transformational Breath® and how it could make her feel. Her first session had been in Florida during a trip.

Mary contacted me to schedule a session because she was having doubts that she could finish writing her book and have it published. And, it was also important that others receive and appreciate the message she intended to convey.

Mary was stuck in a belief system of having to work hard and struggle with most everything in her life. She described herself as "someone who has lived and worked in challenging situations and accepted suffering on the grounds of 'that's life'." So I was excited to know that, if she was willing to follow my guidance and trust the process, her so-called reality could change quickly and easily.

When Mary started breathing, I could see how hard she worked. I suggested she relax more into her body and learn to trust the flow of her breath. As she did, I focused on different points of the body to help her release long-held tensions and old patterns that may have represented suffering and poverty. As her session progressed, I could see her "letting go", in that she was breathing easier and without so much effort. My experience is that as she would start to integrate these old patterns into new possibilities, her life would start to be different. When we completed the session, she was aware that there was now a new potential for her future and how it could flourish.

Mary has left the job where she was overworked and underpaid and has created a situation that gives her the support to finish her book. She has been asked to be a part of a group at Harvard University to share her expertise and was invited to speak at the United Nations. She is full of life and excited for what she will continue to create for her future as she learns to trust her higher self.

Mary's Miracle

"...I am experiencing more personal power and deeper trust in myself. I am more resilient and relaxed in stressful situations, better able to stand up for myself, and to ask for what I want. Most of all, I am no longer willing to suffer in 'boiling frog' type situations. I choose more love, joy and peace in my life. How does the magic work? Well now, who knows? All I can say is that it seems to shift core beliefs and what results from them - which is everything!" And, a publisher is interested in her book!

10.

Self-Worth

Raphael had been dealing with a painful condition called *interstitial cystitis (a chronic painful bladder condition)* for a number of years. By eating a non-acidic diet and taking some medications, he was able to have little or no pain most of the time. Early in 2015, however, Raphael's condition flared up, with some fairly constant pain. He tried tweaking his diet and medication, but was unable to come out of this flare up. After about six months, Raphael decided to try a Transformational Breath session to see if it could help.

I usually ask new clients, "If you could have a miracle today, what would it be?" Raphael elected to be free from pain. Or, to put it in a more empowering format, "I feel WONDERFUL in my body."

When Raphael started breathing, I noticed how shallow his breathing was. This might represent a "closed heart" and a repression of love. At some time in Raphael's past, he unconsciously chose to shut down his heart to protect his feelings. He would get emotional quickly and intensely so we used *toning* (connecting a sound to the essence of the feeling). He began hitting pillows with his hands; this form of physical expression helps move or release the charged energy before we settle back into the breathing cycle.

Working different points of self-love, self-acceptance, and self-compassion seemed to help Raphael relax into a fuller circular breath. One time, he had a memory of a painful breakup, a past that he thought was complete.

After each session, the pain lessened. One particular session brought up another memory, this of his mother having lost a son (Paul) before Raphael was born. His mother believed that Paul was being sent back to her when Raphael was born. When she saw that it wasn't Paul, she was disappointed and Raphael felt that unconscious rejection as an infant.

For years, Raphael had carried the emotional wounds of not being worthy of love by his mother, and by extension, himself. Continued sessions saw him reach the point of being pain-free. He also started to really appreciate and love himself and saw how others in his life responded in that same way.

Raphael's Miracle

He was relieved of the physical pain. And just as important, the more that he felt worthy of love, he noticed the people in his life showing more love to him.

11.

Reclaim Your Superpowers

When Sophia came in for a Transformational Breath session and explained what she wanted to create, I was stunned and thought, "this will take a first class Miracle"... which truth be told, I have seen numerous times. However, this seemed big.

Sophia was studying for her Dental Admissions Test (DAT) to apply to dental school. This test includes four math and science sections, as well as one perceptual ability section. Although Sophia had previously taken courses on these subjects, she needed to relearn them in detail to master the material for the exam.

Specifically, she needed to memorize 2,500 flashcards with different facts for the biology portion of the test that was only five weeks away. She also was taking courses at a nearby university to complete her Bachelor's degree.

As I took a deep breath, I received guidance that stated, "Teach her how powerful she really is."

I work with Miracle Principles (A Course In Miracles Spiritual Text) one of which states "Healing is seeing the spiritual truth of each being's identity." I needed to see Sophia perfectly capable of creating anything she desired.

At Sophia's core, she is... Spirit... a Creator... she is Perfect! My job was to remind her of this and for her to embody her identity and trust that part of herself. From that moment on, I was convinced that Sophia would create her Miracle. My job was merely to help her build a full-connected breath and guide her through any of the blocks that may come up during her sessions.

In this particular session, Sophia had a slight pause between exhaling and inhaling, which could be indicative of,

"Not Accepting Her Own Good". After engaging in some toning and expression, Sophia was easily able to flow into a full open breath. When she completed the session, she knew that she could accomplish this intention.

Sophia not only passed her DAT exam and exceeded her expectations, she believes Transformational Breath has allowed her to recognize how wise and powerful she is. Her "tests proved it"! Sophia knows that she's capable of creating ANYTHING she wishes because she has the power inside her.

Sophia's Miracle

To know without a doubt that she is capable of creating ANYTHING she wishes!

The Transformational Breath Foundation offers an Introductory 2-day Training experience called: ***Reclaim Your Superpowers*** *™.*
www.transformationalbreath.com/pro.aspx

12.

Spiritual Connection

Regina's spiritual evolution was very important to her. Her intention in her Transformational Breath session was to, "Allow her angels and guides to assist her to live from her highest authentic self."

Transformational Breath works on three levels in each session. On the Physical level, it aims to provide more energy in part by opening up restrictive breathing patterns, and enhancing physical health.

On the Mental/Emotional level, Transformational Breath clears old repressed feelings and lower vibrational thoughts and memories, thus creating deeper levels of peace, creativity, and clarity.

And on the third level, the Spiritual, Transformational Breath creates an opening by clearing the lower subconscious, allowing access to higher aspects of self (i.e. superconscious) which is essentially the soul or spiritual dimension. Through *conscious invocation*[1], integration of the spiritual into the physical is accomplished, thereby allowing truer expression of one's spiritual nature.

I focused on being sure that Regina had a full circular breath, where she was breathing into her lower abdomen, solar plexus, and finally up in the high heart area. Regina had a slight pause between exhaling and inhaling and it is important that we eliminate any pause in the breath, as that pause would represent holding onto fear. As a Facilitator, I instructed Regina to breathe continuously in a circular pattern

---

[1] To co-create a desired good by invoking an intention and aligning with Creator Source.

so that as soon as we exhale, we inhale, and as soon as we inhale, we exhale—always connected.

That connection is thought to create a higher vibrational force that is part of the magic of creating the miracles possible with this breathing process. Although, Regina was keeping the breath connected after a little reminder, she started to experience some tightness in her hands, which could be indicative of holding onto something... perhaps a belief or old pattern that could be getting in the way of allowing her to live her highest authentic self. We did some toning (sounding) to release this and allow Regina to just trust and let go of anything that is getting in her way. A beautiful thing about this work is that we don't have to figure out what the emotional content is. We can just state the affirmation silently, "I let go of anything that is in the way of creating my intention" while we continue to breathe. As Regina continued, there was a deeper letting go in her body and a more fluid breath pattern.

When Regina moved into the Spiritual level of her session, she felt that she received two messages from Source (God Energy). The first was to, "look behind your third-eye area" (In yoga, the third-eye refers to the area between and above the eyebrows that leads to inner realms and spaces of higher consciousness), and the other was, "I and My Father are one".

It was interesting that I was wearing a bracelet with those exact words of the latter statement. I felt I was to be passing that message onto someone soon. I knew who that someone was by the end of this session.

Regina was very emotional coming out of her session and felt that she had such a tangible experience of being connected to God and her Angels/Guides. She was also aware of an expansion in her energy field.

Regina's Miracle

To have a palpable experience of being connected to God and her Angels/Guides!

13.

Breath IS Life

When Muriel came for her first Transformational Breath session, the intention was to save a relationship. She was exhausted due to the constant struggle of trying to be comfortable in her *bodymind*[1]. What actually occurred was that Muriel created and maintains a relationship with self.

She had lost her dad from a sudden heart attack, was in a new career coming out of financial hardship, in a troubled relationship and needing to find a new home, all, with no strong support system.

Analyzing Muriel's breath, I could see that she was working really hard, but she was not fully grounded in her body. If we don't have a full lower abdomen when we breathe, it will be difficult to stay really present in our life and create the changes we are hoping for. When we get the breath into the lower abdomen and integrate what is being held there, so much more life energy gets released to use for creation. If we try too hard to get that perfect breath, we create more tension in the body. Compare this to relaxing with a full, easy breath that will allow tension and stress to release from the body. We worked with the breath pattern in Muriel's first couple sessions until it flowed easily and effortlessly.

Her life started to reflect the changes rather quickly. Muriel noticed she didn't feel like she was carrying so much stress and tension. She was getting clear as to what needed to change and what her role was in making the changes. She was willing to come for full breath sessions on a regular basis

---

[1] An approach to understanding the relationship between the human body and the mind in seeing them as a single integrated unit (Wikipedia).

and did her "homework" exercise of a 100 breaths per day to keep her vibration high between sessions.

Muriel is truly creating the life she wants on a regular basis. She knows that when a challenge comes that it can be resolved easily with a breath session. She earns a great living, is able to maintain peaceful and enriching relationships, stays healthy, and is in a new love relationship that works better for her.

Through her practice she truly came to realize that

THE WAY WE BREATHE **IS**
THE WAY WE LIVE OUR LIFE

Muriel's Miracle

To make a lucrative income in real estate in an area where so many are just making it and to have created everything else that is important to her.

14.

Calm Inside The Storm

When Dina first came to see me, she was deep in depression and grief over the loss of her father. She felt like she was living in daily gloom and crying endlessly with no resolution in sight. Upon observing her breath pattern, Dina was holding major tension in her jaw area and not much breath in the abdomen. With the amount of grief that she was carrying, I could understand why it was so difficult for her to stay present in her body, so we started to work with her abdomen.

Our goal was to initiate more of a diaphragmatic breath, because if we didn't fill her lower abdomen to start it would have been difficult to integrate all the emotions she was dealing with. It took a few sessions to bring this about and as she succeeded, the crying episodes let up accordingly. Dina began to feel more alive and able to "show up" in her life.

She also exhibited intense *tetany* [1] in her jaw and hands during early sessions possibly due to holding onto repressed feelings. As she started to express and integrate these feelings, the tetany eased and she felt more open and free.

Dina and I worked consistently for a period of time until she felt truly peaceful and happy. She felt that Transformational Breath gave her vital coping skills and the ability to achieve whatever she needs in her life. She stayed focused on God, creativity and community, found

---

[1] An involuntary steady contraction of muscles that can occur because of significantly decreasing carbon dioxide (CO_2) in the body. This can happen if we breathe too fast or forcefully; essentially the breathing pattern eliminates more CO_2 than the body produces. From an emotional perspective we feel that it often represents a fear pattern.

fearlessness and proved to herself that all challenges could be overcome.

Dina still uses Transformational Breath on her own to keep her vibrations high and to integrate what shows up in her life.

Dina's Miracle

"I firmly believe without the coping skills from my previous Transformational Breath sessions with Kathy, I would have fallen to pieces in the face of the devastation wrought by Hurricane Sandy, in New Jersey, 2012. I was left homeless, and without a job or car.

My life suddenly became incredibly burdensome, but I found myself with the very clear ability to move forward. I took one challenge at a time starting with the most dire, and worked from there. I did not spiral into deep depression. Some days I was sad and frustrated, but it never got so bad that I could not see a way forward. Reflecting often on what I had previously achieved through this incredible Transformational Breath work, I continued in strength, knowing that I would never be so lost as I had once been. It took me years to recover and rebuild my life, but I vowed to myself that I would do it, that I could do it, and that in the end my life would be better than it had ever been.

Now I am very much living that truth. My life circumstances are very happy and healthy. I have what I need to live a joyful life and am supported by self-care and all the good I surround myself with. I have a wonderful living situation, I own my car outright, have dependable employment, and solid foundations on which to build happiness. Kathy and

I meet every so often to continue this journey we started long ago."

Conclusion

I am sharing these stories as a testament to the power of using Transformational Breath and how it can assist us with most anything, especially major events that occur in our lives. Following is a one of those events.

One Monday in 2015 – I remember the day clearly – my sister, Jackie, was rushed to the hospital suffering from heart failure and pneumonia. It shook me to the core, partly because just two days earlier she had left a message, asking me to get in touch. Her message, so calm and peaceful, simply asked me to contact her when I could. No panic, no fear, no clues as to what was brewing.

She never made it back home.

The next few months were stressful, to say the least. Jackie was in a coma for a few weeks and we were told (in Jackie's room where she could hear the conversation) that, due to being without oxygen as a result of the heart failure, she had suffered damage that could not be reversed. The Doctor said not to expect much. The day after this prognosis, she started to come out of the coma and recover.

Then weeks later, we learned that her husband, Bob had stage IV colon and liver cancer and was not offered any treatment options.

Five days later, Jackie had a major stroke and slipped again into a coma.

Her Doctor (in her room) informed us not to expect much. She had major damage to the brain and the best they could offer would be physical therapy if and when she came out of the coma. Again, she responded the next day. That was twice we were told some grim news and twice Jackie started to respond. Was this a coincidence or did Jackie hear the conversation and choose to try to recover and not give up? I believed she was working towards a recovery but Bob was not and soon after, he ended up in the room next to her. Jackie informed her children that, she and their dad had made an agreement - when one of them died, the other would go also. Bob died soon after and Jackie passed the following day.

I was fortunate to be with Jackie at her transition. I did Transformational Breath on a daily basis to help me process the sadness and grief that came up throughout this time. I was then able to stay present and supportive for her and her family throughout this time.

Glossary

Bodymapping – Technique using pressure on various points on the body that are associated with specific emotional content. Putting pressure on these points and breathing can assist us in releasing emotional repressions or physical tensions.

Bodymind – An approach to understanding the relationship between the human body and the mind in seeing them as a single integrated unit (Wikipedia).

Circular Breath – Inhalation and exhalation are connected with no pauses between breaths while breathing with the diaphragm.

Conscious Invocation – To co-create a desired good by invoking an intention and aligning with Creator Source.

Diaphragmatic Breath – Employing the diaphragm muscle during a relaxed inhalation and a relaxed exhalation.

Intention – What we would like to have happen as a result of participating fully in the breath session. This would be something positive and empowering.

Surrender Point – A bodymapping point located beneath the sternum around the *xiphoid process* (bony protrusion) that is usually easy to feel or palpate.

Tetany – An involuntary steady contraction of muscles that can occur because of significantly decreasing carbon dioxide (CO_2) in the body. This can happen if we breathe too fast or forcefully; essentially the breathing pattern eliminates more CO_2 than the body produces. From an emotional perspective we feel that it often represents a fear pattern.

Toning – Using our vocal expression (the power of sound) to help integrate or free energy in the body during the breath session.

Victim Consciousness – A state of consciousness in which we deny personal responsibility for things that happen in our lives or the feelings we experience. We have a belief that the world is against us and we are innocent targets of other people's actions or behavior.

ABOUT KATHY

Kathy Smith is a Certified Transformational Breath Facilitator (CTBF) and Workshop Leader, Naturopathic Doctor, Hypnotherapist, Licensed Massage Therapist, Neuromuscular Therapist, Reiki Master, EMF Practitioner, Professional Level Yoga Teacher, Meditation Teacher, Weight Loss Coach and Life Coach.

With over 20 years of experience in the Holistic Health Field and working with Transformational Breath, Kathy has found Transformational Breath to be the most effective "life changer" for herself and her clients.

Printed in Great Britain
by Amazon